KETO HELPER

I0788086

KETO HELPER

CHRISTINE FARION

Christine Farion

2017

Copyright © 2017 by Christine Farion

All rights reserved. This book or any portion thereof may not be reproduced or used in any manner whatsoever without the express written permission of the publisher except for the use of brief quotations in a book review or scholarly journal.

First Printing: 2017

ISBN 978-1975617233

Christine Farion
Unit 2A, Fulford Business Centre
35 Hospital Fields Road
Fulford, York, UK, YO10 4DZ

www.christinefarion. com

Ordering Information:
Special discounts are available on quantity purchases by corporations, associations, educators, and others. For details, contact the publisher at the above listed address.

U.S. trade bookstores and wholesalers: Please contact Christine Farion via email sales@ilyware.com

CONTENTS

Preface

This handbook was something I needed. I started researching about weight loss, healthy eating and a way to stop my intake of so many sugars!

I was starting to feel very tired by midafternoon and wanted to feel a lot more energetic and alert.

I hope you find some of the information motivational and inspiring and that it helps you stick to your plans. For me, whenever I stray from recording and planning there is correlation with my weight and unhealthy eating going up and up!

This guide is what I use and will continue to use. I couldn't find a guide like it (I did come across some great fitness booklets to record that aspect, which helped me plan aspects in this book) so decided to make one. Having this guide helps remind me of foods, portions, and my macros and I can record when I stray and how to get back on track when I do.

I hope you find it useful – please let me know if you'd like other things added or other fields for information you find important to track.

Thanks!

~ Christine

INTRODUCTION

SUGAR-RICH CARBS are the enemy!

Ok, that may be a little over the top but most of us have been eating the sugar heavy carbs for most of our lives. We don't think about the things we are putting into our body and how it affects us. There is a lot of science research behind the understanding that sugars alter us in several ways but this guide isn't going to explain the basis of Keto. There are already amazing books out there that can do that, as well as a lot of information online.

This is a Keto Helper. If you've decided that Keto is the way for you, and for all the reasons you'll understand: feeling more energetic, having more energy, eating tasty foods, keeping slim, reducing the bad sugary foods we are eating, feeling full for longer and quicker, and many more reasons... then this should be a useful helper guide for you. I will touch a little on the thinking behind Keto and why people choose it in the next chapter.

The book has some of the important basics, which is suitable for someone new to Keto and wanting to understand the basic idea of it – and follow along.

It then has some example foods to eat and what to avoid. There are ideas for menus and some recipes that I make and like. Yes, these are basic but they serve more as a reminder for some of the tasty combinations you might want to try. Most of them are simple to make and won't require specialist equipment or ingredients. I'm happy for you to send me your variations or suggestions as well. You can email me chris@ilyware.com if there are recipes that you have found delicious and easy to make.

There is then the most useful part of the guide and the main purpose; the journal. This is where you can write down your plans for the Keto diet plan and set out your goals for the programme.

CHAPTER 1: WHY KETO?

A KETO DIET is a high-fat, moderate protein, and low – to no- carbohydrate diet. This will encourage the body to stop burning carbohydrates as a primary fuel source, (and protein as the secondary source), and will switch to burning fat. When the body does this, it is entering the state called Ketosis. Low carbohydrate levels cause blood sugar levels to drop and the body begins breaking down fat to use as energy. When this happens, your body becomes incredibly efficient at burning fat for energy. It also turns fat into ketones in the liver, which can supply energy for the brain.

Become a fat burning machine!

Studies show that eating a Keto diet is a proven way to lose weight, in an effective and safe way. The ketogenic diet is suitable for most people and promotes cardiovascular health, stable cholesterol levels as well as mental focus.

Studies have found that maintaining ketosis through a low-carb, low-calorific diet can encourage the body to function more effectively.

There can be a reduction in experiencing energy highs and lows that are triggered by the insulin response that comes with a carbohydrate diet.

It is also important to note that fats are energy high so meals with fats may be a little smaller or you may want to eat less and you will feel fuller.

This is a reason why the food log can be an important tool when doing the Keto diet. It is important to note which foods you are finding filling and what the portions are. If you are trying to lose weight then the calorie count will also become as important as the percentages between the macro distribution.

CHAPTER 2: THE BASICS

In general, the daily intake of net carbs required to enter ketosis could vary from 20to 100 grams per day (and very rarely over 100 grams per day). Most people, who have experienced ketosis, claim to have reached that state at about 20-50 grams of net carbs per day.

There are many things that increase your level of ketosis. Here they are, from most to least important:

Restrict carbohydrates to 20 digestible grams per day or less – a strict low-carb diet. Fiber does not have to be restricted, it might even be beneficial.24

Restrict protein to moderate levels. If possible **stay at or below 1 gram of protein per day, per kg of body weight**. So about 70 grams of protein per day if you weigh 70 kilos (154 pounds). It might be beneficial to lower protein intake even more, especially when overweight, and then aim for 1 gram of protein per kg of desired weight. The most common mistake that stops people from reaching optimal ketosis is too much protein.

Eat enough fat to feel satisfied. This is the big difference between a ketogenic diet and starvation, that also results in ketosis. A ketogenic diet is sustainable, starvation is not.

> If possible stay at or below 1 gram of protein per day, per kg of body weight.
>
> So about 70 grams of protein per day if you weigh 70 kilos.

Avoid snacking when not hungry. Unnecessary snacking slows weight loss and reduces ketosis.

If necessary add intermittent **fasting**, like 16:8. This is very effective at boosting ketone levels, as well as accelerating weight loss and type 2 diabetes reversal.

Add **exercise** – adding any kind of physical activity while on low carb can increase ketone levels moderately. It can also help speed up weight loss and diabetes type 2 reversal slightly. While ketosis is normally safe, it is common to experience some time-limited side effects.

THE FOG

People transitioning from sugar-burning to fat-burning mode often initially experience side effects. This is referred to as the keto flu, since symptoms are like the flu: fatigue, nausea, headaches, cramps, etc. There are two main things that one can do to prevent or alleviate these symptoms:

Drink water with salt and lemon – alternatively have a daily cup of bouillon.

Gradually reduce carbohydrate intake – stopping suddenly results in more temporary symptoms

When starting on a ketogenic diet, you lose water and consequently electrolytes. This is happening since carbs retain water and salts in the body, so when you stop eating carbs your body loses this water. If the keto flu is happening due to too little hydration, it might help to drink a glass of salt water with a little bit of squeezed lemon (for taste).

When carbohydrates are suddenly removed from the diet, the brain can run slightly low on energy before it learns to use ketone bodies for fuel instead of sugar. This means that if you drastically reduce carbs from one day to another, you may get symptoms of such as tiredness, nausea and headaches. Replacing fluids and electrolytes as described above can alleviate the symptoms. Or by instead gradually lowering carb intake over a period of a week or more, the body gets used to burning fat and ketones instead of glucose and there will usually be no symptoms.

CHAPTER 3: MACRONUTRIENTS

Macronutrients are the fuel for the body. There are three 'macros': Fat | Protein | Carbohydrate

> **60% or more of Fats**
>
> **20 – 35% Proteins**
>
> **0 – 5% Carbohydrates**

The carbohydrate count should come from vegetables rather than grains.

The most important thing to reach ketosis is to avoid eating most carbohydrates. You'll probably need to keep carb intake to under 50 grams per day of net carbs, ideally below 20 grams. The fewer carbs the more effective.

This means you'll need to **completely avoid sweet sugary foods**, plus **starchy foods** like bread, pasta, rice and potatoes.

Basically, follow the guidelines for a strict low-carb diet, and remember it's supposed to be high in fat, not high in protein.

A rough guideline is below 10% energy from carbohydrates (the fewer carbs, the more effective), 15-25% protein (the lower end is more effective), and 70% or more from fat.

TOTAL CARBS VS NET CARBS

It is important to keep in mind that some of the foods for the Keto diet are high in fiber. This means that sometimes the digestible ("net") carb content is even lower. To calculate your net carbs, find the carbohydrate count, and then the fiber count:

carbohydrate – fiber = net carbs

The carbs from fiber do not get turned into glucose and is directly removed from the body. Therefore, we don't have to count them in our carb count totals.

CHAPTER 4: LOW CARBS TO ENJOY

You should base most your meals around these foods:

Meat: Red meat, steak, ham, sausage, bacon, chicken and turkey.

Fatty fish: Such as salmon, trout, tuna and mackerel.

Eggs: Look for pastured or omega-3 whole eggs.

Butter and cream: Look for grass-fed when possible.

Cheese: Unprocessed cheese (cheddar, goat, cream, blue or mozzarella).

Nuts and seeds: Almonds, walnuts, flaxseeds, pumpkin seeds, chia seeds, etc.

Healthy oils: Primarily extra virgin olive oil, coconut oil and avocado oil.

Avocados: Whole avocados or freshly made guacamole.

Low-carb veggies: Most green veggies, tomatoes, onions, peppers, etc.

Condiments: You can use salt, pepper and various healthy herbs and spices.

The following pages list other healthy, nutritious and incredibly delicious foods that are suitable.

- Eggs (Almost Zero)

Eggs are among the healthiest and most nutritious foods on the planet. They are loaded with all sorts of nutrients.

All types of meat are close to zero carb. One exception is organ meats like liver, which is about 5% carbs (13).

- Beef (Zero)

Beef is highly satiating and loaded with important nutrients like iron and B12.

- Lamb (Zero)

Lamb tends to be high in a beneficial fatty acid called conjugated linoleic acid, or CLA (14).

- Chicken (Zero)

It is high in many beneficial nutrients, and an excellent source of protein. For low-carb diet, it's a better choice to go for fattier cuts; wings & thighs.

- Pork, Including Bacon (Usually Zero)

Pork is another delicious meat, and bacon is a favorite of many low-carb dieters.

Bacon is a processed meat, so it isn't a "health food." However, it is generally acceptable to eat moderate amounts of bacon on a low-carb diet.

Carbs: read the label and avoid bacon that is cured with sugar.

- Other Low-Carb Meats

Turkey, Veal, Venison

Fish and Seafood

Fish and other seafoods tend to be incredibly nutritious and healthy.

They are particularly high in B12, iodine and omega-3 fatty acids, nutrients many people don't get enough of. Like meat, pretty much all fish and seafood contains next to no carbohydrate.

- Salmon (Zero)

It is a type of fatty fish, meaning that it contains significant amounts of heart-healthy fats, in this case omega-3 fatty acids. Salmon is also loaded with B12, iodine, and contains a decent amount of vitamin D3.

- Trout (Zero)

Like salmon, trout is a type of fatty fish that is loaded with omega-3 fatty acids and other important nutrients.

- Sardines (Zero)

Sardines are oily fish that are generally eaten almost whole, with bones and everything. Sardines are among the most nutrient-dense foods on the planet, and contain almost every single nutrient that the human body needs.

- Shellfish (4-5% Carbs)

Shellfish is among the world's most nutritious foods, ranking close to organ meats when it comes to nutrient density. Shellfish tends to contain small amounts of carbohydrates.

Carbs: 4-5 grams of carbs per 100 grams of shellfish.

- Other Low-Carb Fish and Seafood

Shrimp, Haddock, Herring, Tuna, Cod, Halibut

Vegetables

Most vegetables are low in carbs. Leafy greens are particularly low, with the majority of the carbs in them consisting of fiber.

On the other hand, starchy root vegetables like potatoes and sweet potatoes are high in carbs.

- Broccoli (7%)

Broccoli is a tasty vegetable that can be eaten both raw and cooked. It is high in vitamin C, vitamin K and fiber.

Carbs: 6 grams per cup, or 7 grams per 100 grams.

- Tomatoes (4%)

Tomatoes are technically fruits/berries, but are usually eaten as vegetables. They are high in vitamin C and potassium.

Carbs: 7 grams in a large tomato, or 4 grams per 100 grams.

- Onions (9%)

Onions add powerful flavor to recipes. They are high in fiber, antioxidants and various anti-inflammatory compounds.

Carbs: 11 grams per cup, or 9 grams per 100 grams.

- Brussels Sprouts (7%)

Brussels sprouts are highly nutritious vegetables, related to broccoli and kale. They are very high in vitamin C and vitamin K, and contain numerous beneficial plant compounds.

Carbs: 6 grams per half cup, or 7 grams per 100 grams.

- Cauliflower (5%)

Cauliflower is a tasty and versatile vegetable. It is high in vitamin C, vitamin K and folate.

Carbs: 5 grams per cup, and 5 grams per 100 grams.

- Kale (10%)

Kale is a very popular vegetable among health-conscious individuals. It is loaded with fiber, vitamin C, vitamin K and carotene antioxidants. Kale has numerous health benefits.

Carbs: 7 grams per cup, or 10 grams per 100 grams.

- Eggplant / Aubergene (6%)

Eggplant is another fruit that is commonly consumed as a vegetable. It has many interesting uses, and is very high in fiber.

Carbs: 5 grams per cup, or 6 grams per 100 grams.

- Cucumber (4%)

Cucumber is a popular vegetable with a mild flavor. It consists mostly of water, with a small amount of vitamin K.

Carbs: 2 grams per half cup, or 4 grams per 100 grams.

- Bell Peppers (6%)

Bell peppers are popular fruits/vegetables with a distinct and satisfying flavor. They are very high in fiber, vitamin C and carotene antioxidants.

Carbs: 9 grams per cup, or 6 grams per 100 grams.

- Asparagus (2%)

Asparagus is very high in fiber, vitamin C, folate, vitamin K and carotene antioxidants. It is also very high in protein compared to most vegetables.

Carbs: 3 grams per cup, or 2 grams per 100 grams.

- Green Beans (7%)

Green beans are technically legumes, but they are usually consumed in a similar manner as vegetables. Calorie for calorie, they are extremely high in many nutrients, including fiber, protein, vitamin C, vitamin K, magnesium and potassium.

Carbs: 8 grams per cup, or 7 grams per 100 grams.

- Mushrooms (3%)

Mushrooms technically aren't plants, but edible mushrooms are often categorized as vegetables. They contain decent amounts of potassium, and are high in some B-vitamins.

Carbs: 3 grams per cup, and 3 grams per 100 grams (white mushrooms).

- Other Low-Carb Vegetables

Celery, Spinach, Zucchini, Cabbage

Except for starchy root vegetables, pretty much all vegetables are low in carbs. You can eat a lot of vegetables without going over your carb limit.

FRUITS AND BERRIES

Even though fruits are generally perceived as being healthy, they are highly controversial among low-carbers. That's because most fruits tend to be high in carbs compared to vegetables. Depending on how many carbs you are aiming for, you may want to restrict your fruit intake to 1-2 pieces per day. However, this does not apply to fatty fruits like avocados or olives. Low-sugar berries, such as strawberries, are also excellent.

- Avocado (8.5%)

The avocado is a unique type of fruit. Instead of being high in carbs, it is loaded with healthy fats. Avocados are also extremely high in fiber and potassium, and contain decent amounts of all sorts of other nutrients.

Carbs: 13 grams per cup, or 8.5 grams per 100 grams.

Keep in mind that the majority (about 78%) of the carbs in avocado are fiber, so it contains almost no digestible ("net") carbs.

- Olives (6%)

The olive is another delicious high-fat fruit. It is very high in iron and copper, and contains a decent amount of vitamin E.

Carbs: 2 grams per ounce, or 6 grams per 100 grams.

- Strawberries (8%)

Strawberries are among the lowest carb and most nutrient-dense fruits you can eat. They are very high in vitamin C, manganese and various antioxidants.

Carbs: 11 grams per cup, or 8 grams per 100 grams.

- Apricots (11%)

The apricot is an incredibly delicious fruit. Each apricot contains little carbohydrate, but plenty of vitamin C and potassium.

Carbs: 8 grams in 2 apricots, or 11 grams per 100 grams.

- Other Low-Carb Fruits

Lemons, Kiwi, Oranges, Raspberries

NUTS AND SEEDS

Nuts and seeds are very popular on low-carb diets. They tend to be low in carbs, but high in fat, fiber, protein and various micronutrients. Nuts are often eaten as snacks, but seeds are rather used for adding crunch to salads or recipes. Nut flours and seed flours (such as almond flour, coconut flour and flax seed meal) are also often used to make low-carb breads and other baked foods.

- Almonds (22%)

Almonds are incredibly tasty and crunchy. They are loaded with fiber, vitamin E and are among the world's best sources of magnesium, a mineral that most people don't get enough of. Additionally, almonds are incredibly filling, and have been shown to promote weight loss.

Carbs: 6 grams per ounce, or 22 grams per 100 grams.

- Walnuts (14%)

The walnut is another delicious type of nut. It is particularly high in the omega-3 fatty acid ALA, and contains various other nutrients.

Carbs: 4 grams per ounce, or 14 grams per 100 grams.

- Peanuts (16%)

Peanuts are technically legumes, but tend to be prepared and consumed like nuts. They are very high in fiber, magnesium, vitamin E and various important vitamins and minerals.

Carbs: 5 grams per ounce, or 16 grams per 100 grams.

- Chia Seeds (44%)

Chia seeds are currently among the world's most popular health foods. They are loaded with many important nutrients, and can be used in all sorts of low-carb friendly recipes. Chia seeds are extremely high in fiber, and may be the richest source of dietary fiber on the planet.

Carbs: 12 grams per ounce, or 44 grams per 100 grams.

However, keep in mind that about 86% of the carbs in chia seeds are fiber, so they contain very few digestible ("net") carbs.

- Other Low-Carb Nuts and Seeds

Cashews, Coconuts, Pistachios, Pumpkin seeds, Sunflower seeds

DAIRY

Full-fat dairy products are excellent low-carbohydrate foods. Just make sure to read the label and avoid anything with added sugar.

- Cheese (1.3%)

Cheese is among the tastiest low-carbohydrate foods, and can be eaten both raw and in all sorts of delicious recipes. It goes particularly well with meat, such as on top of a burger (without the bun, of course). Cheese is also highly nutritious. A single thick slice of cheese contains a similar amount of nutrients as an entire glass of milk.

Carbs: 0.4 grams per slice, or 1.3 grams per 100 grams (cheddar).

- Heavy Cream (3%)

Heavy cream contains very little carbohydrate and protein, but is high in dairy fat. Some low-carbers put it in their coffee, or use it in recipes. A bowl of berries with some whipped cream can be a delicious low-carb dessert. I've even used Clotted Cream if I need to balance my macros with more fats. Very delicious!

Carbs: 1 gram per ounce, or 3 grams per 100 grams.

- Full-fat Yogurt (5%)

Full-fat yogurt is exceptionally healthy. It contains many of the same nutrients as whole milk, but yogurt with live cultures is also loaded with beneficial probiotic bacteria.

Carbs: 11 grams per 8 ounce container, or 5 grams per 100 grams.

- Greek Yogurt (4%)

Greek yogurt, also called strained yogurt, is very thick compared to regular yogurt. It is very high in many beneficial nutrients, especially protein.

Carbs: 6 grams per container, or 4 grams per 100 grams.

FATS AND OILS

There are many healthy fats and oils that are acceptable on a low-carb, real food-based diet. Just make sure to avoid refined vegetable oils like soybean oil, corn oil and others, because these are very unhealthy when consumed in excess.

- Butter (Zero)

Once demonized for the high saturated fat content, butter has been making a comeback. Choose grass-fed butter if you can, it is higher in some nutrients.

- Extra Virgin Olive Oil (Zero)

Extra virgin olive oil is the healthiest fat on the planet. It is a staple ingredient on the heart-healthy Mediterranean diet. It is loaded with powerful antioxidants and anti-inflammatory compounds, and has impressive benefits for cardiovascular health.

- Coconut Oil (Zero)

Coconut oil is a very healthy fat, loaded with medium-chain fatty acids that have powerful beneficial effects on metabolism. They have been shown to reduce appetite, boost fat burning and help people lose belly fat.

- Other Low-Carb Friendly Fats

Avocado oil

BEVERAGES

Most sugar-free beverages are perfectly acceptable when eating low-carb. Keep in mind that fruit juices are very high in sugar and carbs, and should be avoided.

- Water

Water should be your go-to beverage, no matter what the rest of your diet consists of.

- Coffee

Despite having been demonized in the past, coffee is very healthy. It is the biggest source of antioxidants in the diet. Just make sure not to add anything unhealthy to your coffee. Black is best, but some full-fat milk or heavy cream is fine as well.

- Tea

Tea, especially green tea, has been studied quite thoroughly and shown to have all sorts of impressive health benefits. It may also boost fat burning slightly.

- Club Soda / Carbonated Water

Club soda is pretty much just water with added carbon dioxide. It is perfectly acceptable as long as there is no sugar in it. Read the label to make sure.

- Dark Chocolate

This may surprise some people, but quality dark chocolate is the perfect low-carb treat. Just make sure to choose real dark chocolate with a 70-85% cocoa content (or higher), then it won't contain much sugar. Dark chocolate has numerous benefits, such as improved brain function and reduced blood pressure. Studies also show that dark chocolate eaters have a much lower risk of heart disease.

Carbs: 13 grams per 1-ounce piece, or 46 grams per 100 grams. This depends on the type, so make sure to read the label.

Keep in mind that about 25% of the carbs in dark chocolate are fiber, so the total digestible carb content is lower.

- Herbs, Spices and Condiments

There is an endless variety of delicious herbs, spices and condiments that you can eat. Most of them are very low in carbs, but pack a powerful nutritional punch and help add flavor to meals.

Some notable examples include salt, pepper, garlic, ginger, cinnamon, mustard and oregano.

SAMPLE MENU

MONDAY

Breakfast: Bacon, eggs and tomatoes.

Lunch: Chicken salad with olive oil and feta cheese.

Dinner: Salmon with asparagus cooked in butter.

TUESDAY

Breakfast: Egg, tomato, basil, cheese omelet.

Lunch: Almond milk, peanut butter, cocoa powder and stevia milkshake.

Dinner: Meatballs, cheddar cheese and vegetables.

WEDNESDAY

Breakfast: A ketogenic milkshake

Lunch: Shrimp salad with olive oil and avocado.

Dinner: Pork chops with Parmesan cheese, broccoli and salad.

THURSDAY

Breakfast: Omelet with avocado, salsa, peppers, onion and spices.

Lunch: A handful of nuts and celery sticks with guacamole and salsa.

Dinner: Chicken stuffed with pesto and cream cheese, along with vegetables.

FRIDAY

Breakfast: Sugar-free yogurt with peanut butter, cocoa powder (and stevia).

Lunch: Beef stir-fry cooked in coconut oil with vegetables.

Dinner: Bun-less burger with bacon, egg and cheese.

SATURDAY

Breakfast: Ham and cheese omelet with vegetables.

Lunch: Ham and cheese slices with nuts.

Dinner: White fish, egg and spinach cooked in coconut oil.

SUNDAY

Breakfast: Poached eggs with bacon and mushrooms.

Lunch: Burger with salsa, cheese and guacamole.

Dinner: Steak and eggs with a side salad.

Chapter 5: High Carbs to Avoid

THE FOLLOWING foods are very high in carbs and sugars. These are some foods to avoid when following a Keto diet.

Sugary foods: Soda, fruit juice, smoothies, cake, ice cream, candy, etc.

Grains or starches: Wheat-based products, rice, pasta, cereal, etc.

Fruit: All fruit, except small portions of berries like strawberries. I have had raspberries with clotted cream to achieve the balance.

Beans or legumes: Peas, kidney beans, lentils, chickpeas, etc.

Root vegetables and tubers: Potatoes, sweet potatoes, carrots, parsnips, etc.

Low-fat or diet products: These are highly processed and often high in carbs.

Some condiments or sauces: These often contain sugar and unhealthy fat. Full fat mayonnaise is 'ok' but ketchup is not.

Unhealthy fat: Limit your intake of processed vegetable oils, mayonnaise, etc.

Alcohol: Due to its carb content, many alcoholic beverages can throw you out of ketosis. If you are having alcohol there are some that are better than others. Cava, Champagne and white wines are at the lower end of the scale, only 2g carbs and low calorie. Grainy beers are at the higher end of carb intake.

Sugar-free diet foods: These are often high in sugar alcohols, which can affect ketone levels in some cases. These foods also tend to be highly processed.

Overall to remember is to avoid carb-based foods like grains, sugars, legumes, rice, potatoes, candy, juice and even most fruits.

Chapter 6: Help! I've strayed from Keto!

THERE MAY be some days when you are out, visiting with friends or family, or just unable to go the low carb route. It happens and it's important to not beat yourself up about it.

Don't panic!

If you find your carb count higher than usual or hitting in the upper ranges, over 50g or so for example, then you may need to make some adjustments to get back into your ketonic state.

Typically, if you have a higher carb day, if you want to quickly get back on the Keto diet, the next day you should **have a fasting day**. This will help to use as much of the sugars as possible, as quickly as possible. This would be done through:

- Eating much later in the day
- Taking on a reduced number of calories (to use up what you've eaten)
- and little to no carbs.

Then just keep on with your Keto diet as usual the following day.

CHAPTER 7: RECIPES AND IDEAS

THESE PAGES have some ideas for combinations, snacks and quick or easy cook meals. I've tried them all and they do all work very well. Feel free to mix it up and add your own combinations of flavors!

IDEAS

There are some great prepared foods that I sometimes grab or have handy in the fridge to balance the macros when needed. Also, to grab for quick snacks or to add to lunches.

- Clotted Cream is a great way to up the fats if needed.
- Snacking Crackling
- Serrano Ham & Manchego Rollitos
- Crispy Bacon Strips
- Sausages
- Double Cream
- Mini Wrapped Cheeses
- Peanut Butter
- Olives or Nuts

CAULIFLOWER PIZZA

This is a single portion, but please note that this is a very filling meal!

INGREDIENTS

- Tomato puree 4 Tbsp
- 2 Tbsp Crème Fresh
- Kalamata Olives (15g) 45 ~
- Steamed Cauliflower 125g
- Almond Flour (optional) ½ cup
- Mozzarella 15g
- Cheddar Cheese 2oz
- Parmesan 1.2oz
- Egg x 1.5 (or 2)
- Herbs, Oregano, Basil etc.

Adjust the toppings for what your pizza preference is. I chose olives but you might prefer to add meats and other cheeses. (Bacon, Chicken, Salami, Hams etc)

This was fun to make and does require some preparation so is a good one at the weekends if you have a little more time.

METHOD

First make the base.

Steam the cauliflower to cook (4-5 minutes).

Once cooked – drain on kitchen towel or a tea towel. You want to remove as much liquid as possible.

Whiz up cauliflower and almond flour if using in a food processor

In a bowl, combine the cauliflower mix with the mozzarella, Parmesan, oregano, salt, garlic powder and eggs.

Transfer to the center of the baking sheet (lined with baking parchment or a non-stick surface) and spread into a circle, resembling a pizza crust. You can make the 'edges' a little higher like on a typical pizza crust.

Bake for 20 minutes, or until golden.

Mix crème fresh and tomato puree. Spread thinly on the base of the pizza.

Add desired toppings and bake an additional 10 minutes.

Tip: Make one for now, and save one for later. After baking the crusts and adding the toppings, wrap up the whole pizza in foil, and FREEZE it for a quick "frozen pizza" to enjoy another night! Simply thaw and bake until the cheese is hot and bubbly!

COCONUT FLATBREAD

These are nice formed into the shape you want (square, rectangle, etc.) and then you can use it for sandwiches or to put eggs on top and similar.

I also added a small amount of Psyllium Husk for fiber (half a teaspoon).

INGREDIENTS

- 1 1/2 Tablespoons coconut flour
- 1 Tablespoon coconut oil, melted
- 1 Egg
- 1/8 Teaspoon sea salt (a sprinkle)
- 1/4 Teaspoon Baking Powder

METHOD

Preheat oven to 350 degrees.

Mix coconut flour, sea salt, and baking powder together until combined.

Add egg and melted coconut oil and mix well.

Let batter sit for a few minutes to allow the flour to absorb the liquid.

Scoop half the batter on baking pan and use a spatula to spread batter into a circle the size of a bun.

Repeat using the rest of the batter. Bake for 10 minutes or until golden brown.

Parmesan Chips

Delicious snack! Quick and easy to make. Be warned about the surface you cook these on because they might stick! I like to keep some saved as snacks or make extra for friends to enjoy.

Measure out your parmesan to work out your macros. 2.5oz of cheese is around 2g carbs, 17g fat, 27g protein and 275 calories.

Ingredients

- Parmesan - several ounces
- Maybe a dip? Sour cream or similar

Method

Heat your oven to 200

Grate the parmesan, I've grated it both on the finer setting and the thicker one and results are similar so it's up to you.

Line a baking sheet with grease proof paper or use a non-stick pan.

Make small piles of cheese spread out on the pan. You might get 9-12 per baking sheet.

Cook carefully – they can burn quickly. You will probably want to watch them.

(Other) If you leave it for a little longer they become thinner and a little crunchier. If you take them out just as they brown, the centers are a little soft and edges crunchy which makes a tasty snack.

CAULIFLOWER MASH & STEAK

This is a great Friday night dinner. It always feels a real treat eating this.

INGREDIENTS

- Cauliflower
- Steak
- Oil
- Butter
- Cheese of your choice, strong Cheddar works well
- Seasoning

METHOD

Prepare the cauliflower mash first & keep warm. Remove your steak from the fridge.

Cut the cauliflower into small pieces and steam or boil.

Once cooked, drain the cauliflower.

Add the ingredients according to your macros, if you need more fats you may want more butter for example. Add butter and cheese.

Mash. I mashed with a fork to keep it a little less refined but the choice is yours. Season.

Heat a frying pan

Rub steak with oil, season & fry

Serve!

BOILED COD & BUTTER

This is a very easy meal to make. If you just cook it slow enough the cod just falls apart perfectly.

INGREDIENTS

- Cod
- Lemon
- Milk or Water to boil the cod in
- Butter 1 Tbsp.
- Parsley
- Spinach
- Parmesan

METHOD

Heat some water or milk in a deep frying pan.

Gently place the Cod in the simmering liquid, cover (if possible with a clear lid)

Cook for around 10 minutes. Your time will vary depending on how thick the fish is. You want it just cooked, not overdone.

Cook spinach, this can be put into a pan, or micro-waved. Do not overcook.

Place spinach on plate, sprinkle parmesan on top

Remove fish and drain, it will be delicate so go carefully with it

Place on top of the spinach & parmesan

Rub the hot fish with 1 tbsp of butter to melt it into the fish. Season and add lemon to taste.

PARMESAN ENCRUSTED PORK FILET

This is a great dish for the whole family. You can add potatoes or similar for other family members. Or cauliflower mash!

INGREDIENTS

- 1 x 70g (2½oz) pack rocket
- 3-4 tbsp olive oil
- ½ lemon
- 1½tsp capers, drained and roughly chopped
- 100g (3½oz) Pork rinds crushed
- 25g (1oz) Parmesan cheese
- 1 egg, beaten
- almond flour, for dusting
- 660g (1lb 5oz) pack thin-cut pork steaks

METHOD

Put the rocket into a food processor along with 2 tbsp olive oil and a squeeze of lemon juice.

Whizz together until it forms a rough paste.

Stir in the capers then set aside.

Mix the crushed pork rinds and Parmesan together on a wide plate.

Pour the egg into a large, shallow bowl. Pat the meat dry with kitchen paper, season well and dust with almond flour.

Dip each steak into the beaten egg and then press into the rinds and cheese mixture until they are coated all over.

Heat a little of the olive oil in a large pan. Cook the crumbed steaks for 3-5 minutes on each side, until the coating is golden and crisp and the meat cooked through (you might find it easier to do this in batches).

Serve with a dollop of the rocket dressing.

SALMON FILETS ON SPINACH

Slam up the heat on your oven, cook for 10 minutes and it's perfect!

INGREDIENTS

- Salmon Filets
- Spinach
- Parmesan
- Lemon

METHOD

Heat your oven to maximum temperature.

Place the salmon filets on a baking tray and put into the hot oven.

Cook for 10 minutes, but watch the filets as your oven may differ. It may take a minute or two more or less.

Cook your spinach, place on plate.

Cover with grated Parmaesan

Place the filets on top.

Dress with salt and lemon.

BOILED EGGS & SOY SAUCE

This is a great quick lunch meal, super tasty too!

INGREDIENTS

- 2 Eggs
- 6ml Soy Sauce (half a table spoon)

METHOD

Boil your eggs for 5-6 minutes if you like them soft boiled, longer for hard boiled.

When cooked, take off the heat, and pour cold water on the egg. Leave the eggs in cold water until ready to eat.

Crack egg top and add soy sauce.

(Other) I saw a recipe for boiling eggs which worked well. When the water is boiling, turn the heat to very low. Place the egg gently in it and keeping the heat very low put a lid on the pan. Leave for 6 minutes. Drain and rinse in cold water.

CHICKEN TAGINE STYLE

This is such a flavorful dish!

INGREDIENTS

- Chicken thighs, skin on
- Coconut oil
- Onion
- Coriander fresh for garnish
- Ground Coriander 1 tsp
- Saffron a few strands
- Turmeric 1 tsp
- Chicken Stock

METHOD

Boil a kettle and make the chicken stock. Add saffron strands.

Heat your oil and when hot, place the chicken thighs skin side down into the hot oil.

Cook for around 10 minutes until all the skin is very crispy.

Remove the chicken from the pan and set aside.

Cook the onions until they become clear.

Add your spices and stir constantly for a minute or so. Then add the chicken back in.

Pour in the stock, bring to the boil then simmer for 20-30 minutes, until chicken is cooked.

Prawns, Cheddar & Butter

This isn't so much a recipe as an idea for a snack or to add if you need altering your macros.

Warm the prawns, and fry lightly in butter. When hot through, sprinkle the cheese on top and stir until melted. Serve!

Nut Butter

This can be done with different nuts. You can make your own Almond Butter which will have no preservatives and cost far less than at the supermarkets.

Roast the nuts in the oven. Roast for 12 -15 minutes or so, turning over halfway and roast the other side.

Place roasted nuts into a food processor. It will begin to powder, then clump over time. You will need to scrape the sides of the food processor with a spatula. This process may take around 12 minutes.

Add any flavors you'd like. Ideas are cinnamon, vanilla, honey etc.

This will store in the cupboard for many months. Try spreading on an apple!

OMELETS

This is an idea of what you might like to try as an alternative way to eat eggs. Mix eggs with a little cream to make it a little fluffier and add in your ingredients. You might like to try some of the following:

Cheese, cheddar, parmesan, Red Leicester... try in the omelet and on top.

Meats, hams, bacon

Mushrooms, peppers, spinach

Herbs, parsley, chives

LETTUCE WRAPPED BURGER

This is listed here as an idea. I've enjoyed bar-b-q's where the burgers were cooked and then I placed it on a salad or wrap it in lettuce! A great carb free option.

If you're making the burgers, try putting cheese in the middle!

Duck with Pak Choi

This is incredibly tasty and easy to make. It looks great too!

Ingredients

- 4 duck breasts, skin on and trimmed of any excess fat
- 1tsp five-spice powder
- salt
- pepper
- 4 pak choi, whole with the bottom end trimmed
- 100g shiitake mushrooms, sliced
- 1 small carrot, finely sliced
- 1tbsp sesame seeds
- 1l chicken stock
- 2tbsp dark soy sauce
- 2tbsp sesame oil
- 2 cloves garlic, roughly chopped
- coriander, to garnish

Method

Preheat the oven to 200°C.

Make slashes through the skin and fat of the duck breasts and rub all over with the five-spice powder and season with salt and pepper.

Heat a heavy frying pan over a medium flame and place the duck breasts skin side down. Fry for 4-5 minutes until the skin is golden and crispy and turn over so the skin side is facing up.

Transfer to the oven for 8-10 minutes or until the duck breasts feel firm yet springy to the touch.

Meanwhile, bring the chicken stock and soy sauce to the boil in a large saucepan and then add the pak choi, garlic, mushrooms and carrot.

Turn the heat down and simmer gently for a few minutes. Remove the duck from the oven and let it rest for 5 minutes. Slice the duck breasts evenly.

Arrange the broth in bowls and top with the duck breasts on top and garnish with the sesame seeds and sprigs of coriander.

CHICKEN KORMA

You might want to make a coconut or almond flat bread to eat this with.

INGREDIENTS

- 4 skinless chicken breasts, diced
- 50ml oil, Olive or coconut
- 2 cloves garlic, minced
- 1 onion, finely chopped
- 1 inch piece of ginger, minced
- 1/2 teaspoon chilli powder
- 1/2 teaspoon ground cinnamon
- 1/2 teaspoon ground turmeric
- 1/2 teaspoon ground white pepper
- 150ml passata (about 7g of carbs)
- 130ml chicken stock
- 2 tablespoons ground almonds
- 4 tablespoons double cream
- 4 tablespoons plain yogurt
- salt
- pepper
- parsley leaves, to garnish

METHOD

Sweat the onion, garlic and ginger in a large casserole dish over a medium heat for 5-6 minutes until soft, stirring occasionally.

Add all the spices and continue to cook for 1-2 minutes, stirring occasionally.

Add the passata and chicken stock and bring to a simmer.

Stir in the ground almonds and the chicken and simmer for 10-12 minutes until the chicken is cooked with no pink showing.

Stir in the cream and yogurt and adjust the seasoning to taste.

PANCETTA WRAPPED CHICKEN

Or swap for pancetta wrapped Salmon

INGREDIENTS

- 4 chicken breast fillets
- 250g ball mozzarella, sliced into 8
- 20g basil
- 80g Parma ham
- 1tsp olive oil

METHOD

Preheat the oven to gas 6, 200°C, fan 180°C. Lay out the fillets on a board.

Season all over and make a small incision about 4–5cm long and 3cm deep in the middle of each one.

Stuff 2 slices of the mozzarella and 3 basil leaves into the 'pocket' – don't worry if either is poking out a little.

Wrap each chicken breast with 1 1/2 slices of the Parma ham to conceal the pocket.

Heat the oil in a pan and sear on both sides until golden.

Place on a roasting tray and bake in the oven for 15-20 minutes, until the chicken is cooked with no pink showing.

BACON & EGGS

Just to remind you of the classic breakfasts.

INGREDIENTS

- Bacon
- Eggs

METHOD

Add bacon to pan, fry until ready.

Put the bacon on a plate, fry a few eggs (I use 3-4) in the bacon fat.

(Optional) If you want to add some flavor to the eggs, put a bit of sea salt, garlic powder and onion powder on them while frying.

Chicken in creamy mushroom Sauce

A saucy dish!

Ingredients

- 15g (1/2 oz) dried wild mushrooms
- 1 tbsp olive oil
- 15g (1/2oz) butter
- 4 chicken breasts, skin on
- 1 large onion, finely sliced
- 2 garlic cloves, chopped
- 250g (8oz) chestnut mushrooms, sliced
- 200ml (1/3pt) hot chicken stock
- 1/2x30g pack fresh tarragon leaves, picked and chopped
- 200g (7oz) creme fraiche

Method

In a small bowl, soak the dried mushrooms in boiling water for 15 minutes.

Strain and save the liquid. Chop the mushrooms and set aside.

Meanwhile, heat the olive oil and butter in a large frying pan over a medium-high heat. Season the chicken on both sides and then fry for 5 minutes, skin side down.

Turn the breasts over and fry for another 3-4 minutes. Remove from the pan and set aside.

Add the onion and fry for 3-4 minutes. Then mix in the chestnut mushrooms and fry for a further 3 minutes.

Add the garlic and reserved chopped mushrooms and fry for 1 minute.

Pour in 100ml of the mushroom soaking liquid and the hot stock and two thirds of the chopped tarragon. Return the browned chicken pieces to the pan.

Bring to the boil then turn down the heat and simmer for 10 minutes or until the chicken is cooked.

Stir in the crème fraîche and warm through but don't boil.

Scatter over the rest of the tarragon.

Spring roasted chicken with Tarragon

This is delicious. One of my favorite ways to cook a roast chicken.

Ingredients

- 1 whole chicken, about 1.3kg (2.9lb)
- 25g (1oz) unsalted butter, softened
- 1 x 30g pack fresh tarragon
- a sprig of fresh thyme
- 200ml white wine
- 1 x 300g bag shallots, peeled
- 1 bulb of garlic
- 175g unsmoked bacon
- 150g (5oz) peas, defrosted if frozen or blanched if fresh

Method

Preheat the oven Gas 5, 190°C, 375°F. Put the chicken in a roasting tray. Smear the butter all over and season well.

Put a large sprig of the tarragon and the thyme into the cavity and pour the wine around, adding a splash of water as well.

Roast for 30mins, then add the whole shallots, bacon and garlic to the tin. Roast for another 40mins, adding a splash more water if the juices in the roasting tray dry up.

Lift the chicken with some tongs so the juices run from the cavity. The chicken is cooked if the juices are clear - if they're still slightly pink, cook for a further 10mins.

Stir the peas into the juices around the bird and scatter with some fresh tarragon. Allow to sit for 10mins, then remove from the roasting tin and carve.

Reduce the juices a little to make some gravy and serve with new potatoes and vegetables or salad.

Cooking tip

If you've got leftover chicken, turn it into a tasty and quick chicken salad. Shred the meat and toss it together with mixed salad leaves. Just before serving, dress it with extra virgin olive oil and lemon juice.

ALMOND QUICHE

This is a nice take on a quiche.

INGREDIENTS

- 2 Cups Almond flour
- ½ Cup melted butter
- 1 Tbsp garlic
- ½ tsp salt / pepper

For the filling

- 8 oz button mushrooms
- 1 clove garlic, mince
- 10 oz box frozen spinach, thawed
- 4 large eggs
- 1 cup full-fat milk or cream
- 2 oz feta cheese
- Other cheese, Swiss etc
- ¼ cup Parmesan, grated
- ½ cup shredded mozzarella
- (Bacon bits optional)

METHOD

Preheat oven to 350 degrees F (175 degrees C).

Mix almond meal, butter, garlic, 1/2 teaspoon sea salt, and 1/8 teaspoon white pepper together, forming a ball. Gently press dough into a 9-inch pie pan.

Bake crust in the preheated oven for 10 minutes. The crust will puff up slightly; gently press it back down with a spoon or fork. Continue baking until just lightly browned, 8 to 10 minutes.

Squeeze the excess moisture from the thawed spinach. Rinse any dirt or debris from the mushrooms, then slice thinly. Mince the garlic.

Add the mushrooms, garlic, and a pinch of salt and pepper to a non-skillet spritzed lightly with non-stick spray (or a splash of cooking oil).

Sauté the mushrooms and garlic until the mushrooms are soft and all of their moisture has evaporated away (5-7 minutes).

If using, sprinkle bacon into the bottom of the pie crust.

Place the squeeze-dried spinach in the bottom of the pie dish.

Place the sautéed mushrooms on top of the spinach, followed by the crumbled feta.

In a medium bowl, whisk together the eggs, milk, and Parmesan. Season lightly with pepper.

Pour the egg mixture over the vegetables and feta in the pie dish. Top with the shredded mozzarella.

Place the pie dish on a baking sheet for easy transfer in and out of the oven.

Bake in the preheated oven until a knife inserted in the center comes out clean, about 35 minutes. , Or until the top is golden brown (ovens may vary). Let cool for 5 to 10 minutes to finish setting in the middle. Cut into 6 slices.

BROCCOLI CHEESE SOUP

An idea for cold winters. Around 6 servings.

Calories: 353, Total Carbohydrates: 7g, Fiber: 3g,
Net Carbohydrates: 4g, Protein: 8g, Fat 10g.

INGREDIENTS

- 2 tablespoons butter
- 1 ½ cups heavy cream
- 2 ½ cups water (for a thicker soup – add less)
- chicken broth — about 4 cups
- ¾ teaspoon salt
- ½ teaspoon dry mustard
- ¼ teaspoon cayenne pepper
- 16oz frozen chopped broccoli — thawed and drained
- ½ cup red bell pepper — finely chopped
- 8 oz shredded cheddar cheese — strong or extra strong
- 2 Tbsp chopped chives

METHOD

Melt butter in a large saucepan over medium heat. Cook and stir 30 seconds or until bubbly.

Add cream, water, broth, salt, mustard and cayenne pepper; bring to a simmer over high heat, stirring frequently.

Add broccoli and red pepper; return to a boil. Reduce heat to low; simmer uncovered 5 minutes, stirring occasionally.

Add cheese; stir over low heat just until cheese melts (do not boil). Top with chives if desired.

CHAPTER 8: USING THE JOURNAL

I USE my journal as my planner. It helps me **to plan** one week at a time, and to buy the ingredients necessary for the week.

BUDGET MONEY AND CARBS!

Using a journal, I can budget to understand roughly what carbs and calories I'll be eating. I use it as a guide – I can deviate from it if there is something else happening that day or night. I may plan some alcohol for example so I'd make sure I had little to no carbs earlier in the day. The important thing to note is that when I plan and buy the food that is needed for my menu – it is a lot easier to stick to it and reach your goals.

For example; lunches at work are too often a quick grab from a local shop. Planning eliminates those unhealthy calorie-high foods. People tend to grab a sandwich, crisps or chocolate bar for a quick food hit but if you were to plan for your lunch – you'd probably choose something else.

During the week, I'll weigh out the portions and put them into an app (My Fitness Pal is the one I use) to make sure I hit the macros I'm after. This works well for me and I scan a lot of the barcodes on the products to get the accurate information.

Use the journal how it suits you. Here is how I use mine:

Weekly Goal:

In this section I tend to put a goal that may be weight loss, amount of coffee or water and similar. I note the goal, how I can achieve it, and what reward I could get if I reach it.

Fitness Goal:

Keeping fit is an important aspect of everyone's lives. I've put a space here for fitness goals because I know I can lapse a bit on this unless it's a bit more in my face. I like to set a weekly goal. This could be the amount of time every day that you'd like to spend, or more generic, such as do a 2 mile walk every day.

Reflection:

This is the place that I can come to at the start of a week and reflect on what went well and what didn't. I may have gained weight, or stayed standing at the same weight and so it can be useful to understand why. I also reflect on how often I eat out versus a home cooked meal. This is your place to reflect on the week and what went right, what should you stop doing, what should you change doing and what should you continue doing.

Calendar Portion:

I'll write in what I'm planning of doing so I am able to plan the week in a general way. This helps me shop for ingredients and work in if I have plans on an evening or similar where I may not be able to work through a keto diet.

Christine Farion

PERSONAL JOURNAL
Weeks 1-4

Weekly Goal:
Goal | Plan of Action | Reward

Fitness Goal:

Reflection:

MONDAY		Carbs | Fats | Proteins | Calories
TOTAL Ca= Fa= Pr= Cals=	Breakfast	
	Lunch	
	Dinner	

TUESDAY		Carbs | Fats | Proteins | Calories
TOTAL Ca= Fa= Pr= Cals=	Breakfast	
	Lunch	
	Dinner	

WEDS		Carbs | Fats | Proteins | Calories
TOTAL Ca= Fa= Pr= Cals=	Breakfast	
	Lunch	
	Dinner	

THURSDAY		Carbs | Fats | Proteins | Calories
TOTAL Ca= Fa= Pr= Cals=	Breakfast	
	Lunch	

	Dinner	

FRIDAY		*Carbs | Fats | Proteins | Calories*
TOTAL Ca= Fa= Pr= Cals=	Breakfast	
	Lunch	
	Dinner	

SATURDAY		*Carbs | Fats | Proteins | Calories*
TOTAL Ca= Fa= Pr= Cals=	Breakfast	
	Lunch	
	Dinner	

SUNDAY		*Carbs | Fats | Proteins | Calories*
TOTAL Ca= Fa= Pr= Cals=	Breakfast	
	Lunch	
	Dinner	

MONDAY		Carbs | Fats | Proteins | Calories
TOTAL Ca= Fa= Pr= Cals=	Breakfast	
	Lunch	
	Dinner	

TUESDAY		Carbs | Fats | Proteins | Calories
TOTAL Ca= Fa= Pr= Cals=	Breakfast	
	Lunch	
	Dinner	

WEDS		Carbs | Fats | Proteins | Calories
TOTAL Ca= Fa= Pr= Cals=	Breakfast	
	Lunch	
	Dinner	

THURSDAY		Carbs | Fats | Proteins | Calories
TOTAL Ca= Fa= Pr= Cals=	Breakfast	
	Lunch	

	Dinner	

FRIDAY		*Carbs	Fats	Proteins	Calories*
TOTAL Ca= Fa= Pr= Cals=	Breakfast	
	Lunch	
	Dinner	

SATURDAY		*Carbs	Fats	Proteins	Calories*
TOTAL Ca= Fa= Pr= Cals=	Breakfast	
	Lunch	
	Dinner	

SUNDAY		*Carbs	Fats	Proteins	Calories*
TOTAL Ca= Fa= Pr= Cals=	Breakfast	
	Lunch	
	Dinner	

MONDAY		Carbs | Fats | Proteins | Calories
TOTAL Ca= Fa= Pr= Cals=	Breakfast	
	Lunch	
	Dinner	

TUESDAY		Carbs | Fats | Proteins | Calories
TOTAL Ca= Fa= Pr= Cals=	Breakfast	
	Lunch	
	Dinner	

WEDS		Carbs | Fats | Proteins | Calories
TOTAL Ca= Fa= Pr= Cals=	Breakfast	
	Lunch	
	Dinner	

THURSDAY		Carbs | Fats | Proteins | Calories
TOTAL Ca= Fa= Pr= Cals=	Breakfast	
	Lunch	

	Dinner	

FRIDAY		*Carbs | Fats | Proteins | Calories*
TOTAL Ca= Fa= Pr= Cals=	Breakfast	
	Lunch	
	Dinner	

SATURDAY		*Carbs | Fats | Proteins | Calories*
TOTAL Ca= Fa= Pr= Cals=	Breakfast	
	Lunch	
	Dinner	

SUNDAY		*Carbs | Fats | Proteins | Calories*
TOTAL Ca= Fa= Pr= Cals=	Breakfast	
	Lunch	
	Dinner	

MONDAY		Carbs | Fats | Proteins | Calories
TOTAL Ca= Fa= Pr= Cals=	Breakfast	
	Lunch	
	Dinner	

TUESDAY		Carbs | Fats | Proteins | Calories
TOTAL Ca= Fa= Pr= Cals=	Breakfast	
	Lunch	
	Dinner	

WEDS		Carbs | Fats | Proteins | Calories
TOTAL Ca= Fa= Pr= Cals=	Breakfast	
	Lunch	
	Dinner	

THURSDAY		Carbs | Fats | Proteins | Calories
TOTAL Ca= Fa= Pr= Cals=	Breakfast	
	Lunch	

	Dinner	

FRIDAY		*Carbs	Fats	Proteins	Calories*
TOTAL Ca= Fa= Pr= Cals=	Breakfast	
	Lunch	
	Dinner	

SATURDAY		*Carbs	Fats	Proteins	Calories*
TOTAL Ca= Fa= Pr= Cals=	Breakfast	
	Lunch	
	Dinner	

SUNDAY		*Carbs	Fats	Proteins	Calories*
TOTAL Ca= Fa= Pr= Cals=	Breakfast	
	Lunch	
	Dinner	

4- WEEK INTERVAL

Take time to assess your goals and progress. How is the program working for you?

Goals Set

Goals Reached

Set New Targets

Assess the last 4 weeks

Personal Journal
Continuing, Weeks 5-8

Weekly Goal:
Goal | Plan of Action | Reward

Fitness Goal:

Reflection:

MONDAY		Carbs | Fats | Proteins | Calories
TOTAL Ca= Fa= Pr= Cals=	Breakfast	
	Lunch	
	Dinner	

TUESDAY		Carbs | Fats | Proteins | Calories
TOTAL Ca= Fa= Pr= Cals=	Breakfast	
	Lunch	
	Dinner	

WEDS		Carbs | Fats | Proteins | Calories
TOTAL Ca= Fa= Pr= Cals=	Breakfast	
	Lunch	
	Dinner	

THURSDAY		Carbs | Fats | Proteins | Calories
TOTAL Ca= Fa= Pr= Cals=	Breakfast	
	Lunch	

	Dinner	

FRIDAY		*Carbs | Fats | Proteins | Calories*
TOTAL Ca= Fa= Pr= Cals=	Breakfast	
	Lunch	
	Dinner	

SATURDAY		*Carbs | Fats | Proteins | Calories*
TOTAL Ca= Fa= Pr= Cals=	Breakfast	
	Lunch	
	Dinner	

SUNDAY		*Carbs | Fats | Proteins | Calories*
TOTAL Ca= Fa= Pr= Cals=	Breakfast	
	Lunch	
	Dinner	

MONDAY		Carbs | Fats | Proteins | Calories
TOTAL Ca= Fa= Pr= Cals=	Breakfast	
	Lunch	
	Dinner	

TUESDAY		Carbs | Fats | Proteins | Calories
TOTAL Ca= Fa= Pr= Cals=	Breakfast	
	Lunch	
	Dinner	

WEDS		Carbs | Fats | Proteins | Calories
TOTAL Ca= Fa= Pr= Cals=	Breakfast	
	Lunch	
	Dinner	

THURSDAY		Carbs | Fats | Proteins | Calories
TOTAL Ca= Fa= Pr= Cals=	Breakfast	
	Lunch	

	Dinner	

FRIDAY — *Carbs | Fats | Proteins | Calories*

TOTAL Ca= Fa= Pr= Cals=	Breakfast	
	Lunch	
	Dinner	

SATURDAY — *Carbs | Fats | Proteins | Calories*

TOTAL Ca= Fa= Pr= Cals=	Breakfast	
	Lunch	
	Dinner	

SUNDAY — *Carbs | Fats | Proteins | Calories*

TOTAL Ca= Fa= Pr= Cals=	Breakfast	
	Lunch	
	Dinner	

MONDAY		Carbs | Fats | Proteins | Calories
TOTAL Ca= Fa= Pr= Cals=	Breakfast	
	Lunch	
	Dinner	

TUESDAY		Carbs | Fats | Proteins | Calories
TOTAL Ca= Fa= Pr= Cals=	Breakfast	
	Lunch	
	Dinner	

WEDS		Carbs | Fats | Proteins | Calories
TOTAL Ca= Fa= Pr= Cals=	Breakfast	
	Lunch	
	Dinner	

THURSDAY		Carbs | Fats | Proteins | Calories
TOTAL Ca= Fa= Pr= Cals=	Breakfast	
	Lunch	

	Dinner	

FRIDAY		*Carbs	Fats	Proteins	Calories*
TOTAL Ca= Fa= Pr= Cals=	Breakfast	
	Lunch	
	Dinner	

SATURDAY		*Carbs	Fats	Proteins	Calories*
TOTAL Ca= Fa= Pr= Cals=	Breakfast	
	Lunch	
	Dinner	

SUNDAY		*Carbs	Fats	Proteins	Calories*
TOTAL Ca= Fa= Pr= Cals=	Breakfast	
	Lunch	
	Dinner	

MONDAY		Carbs | Fats | Proteins | Calories
TOTAL Ca= Fa= Pr= Cals=	Breakfast	
	Lunch	
	Dinner	

TUESDAY		Carbs | Fats | Proteins | Calories
TOTAL Ca= Fa= Pr= Cals=	Breakfast	
	Lunch	
	Dinner	

WEDS		Carbs | Fats | Proteins | Calories
TOTAL Ca= Fa= Pr= Cals=	Breakfast	
	Lunch	
	Dinner	

THURSDAY		Carbs | Fats | Proteins | Calories
TOTAL Ca= Fa= Pr= Cals=	Breakfast	
	Lunch	

| | Dinner | |

FRIDAY		*Carbs | Fats | Proteins | Calories*
TOTAL Ca= Fa= Pr= Cals=	Breakfast	
	Lunch	
	Dinner	

SATURDAY		*Carbs | Fats | Proteins | Calories*
TOTAL Ca= Fa= Pr= Cals=	Breakfast	
	Lunch	
	Dinner	

SUNDAY		*Carbs | Fats | Proteins | Calories*
TOTAL Ca= Fa= Pr= Cals=	Breakfast	
	Lunch	
	Dinner	

4- Week Interval

Take time to assess your goals and progress. How is the program working for you?

Goals Set

Goals Reached

Set New Targets

Assess the last 4 weeks

PERSONAL JOURNAL
Continuing, Weeks 9-12

Weekly Goal:
Goal | Plan of Action | Reward

Fitness Goal:

Reflection:

MONDAY		Carbs | Fats | Proteins | Calories
TOTAL Ca= Fa= Pr= Cals=	Breakfast	
	Lunch	
	Dinner	

TUESDAY		Carbs | Fats | Proteins | Calories
TOTAL Ca= Fa= Pr= Cals=	Breakfast	
	Lunch	
	Dinner	

WEDS		Carbs | Fats | Proteins | Calories
TOTAL Ca= Fa= Pr= Cals=	Breakfast	
	Lunch	
	Dinner	

THURSDAY		Carbs | Fats | Proteins | Calories
TOTAL Ca= Fa= Pr= Cals=	Breakfast	
	Lunch	

	Dinner	

FRIDAY		*Carbs | Fats | Proteins | Calories*
TOTAL Ca= Fa= Pr= Cals=	Breakfast	
	Lunch	
	Dinner	

SATURDAY		*Carbs | Fats | Proteins | Calories*
TOTAL Ca= Fa= Pr= Cals=	Breakfast	
	Lunch	
	Dinner	

SUNDAY		*Carbs | Fats | Proteins | Calories*
TOTAL Ca= Fa= Pr= Cals=	Breakfast	
	Lunch	
	Dinner	

MONDAY		Carbs | Fats | Proteins | Calories
TOTAL Ca= Fa= Pr= Cals=	Breakfast	
	Lunch	
	Dinner	

TUESDAY		Carbs | Fats | Proteins | Calories
TOTAL Ca= Fa= Pr= Cals=	Breakfast	
	Lunch	
	Dinner	

WEDS		Carbs | Fats | Proteins | Calories
TOTAL Ca= Fa= Pr= Cals=	Breakfast	
	Lunch	
	Dinner	

THURSDAY		Carbs | Fats | Proteins | Calories
TOTAL Ca= Fa= Pr= Cals=	Breakfast	
	Lunch	

	Dinner	

FRIDAY		*Carbs	Fats	Proteins	Calories*
TOTAL Ca= Fa= Pr= Cals=	Breakfast	
	Lunch	
	Dinner	

SATURDAY		*Carbs	Fats	Proteins	Calories*
TOTAL Ca= Fa= Pr= Cals=	Breakfast	
	Lunch	
	Dinner	

SUNDAY		*Carbs	Fats	Proteins	Calories*
TOTAL Ca= Fa= Pr= Cals=	Breakfast	
	Lunch	
	Dinner	

MONDAY		Carbs | Fats | Proteins | Calories
TOTAL Ca= Fa= Pr= Cals=	Breakfast	
	Lunch	
	Dinner	

TUESDAY		Carbs | Fats | Proteins | Calories
TOTAL Ca= Fa= Pr= Cals=	Breakfast	
	Lunch	
	Dinner	

WEDS		Carbs | Fats | Proteins | Calories
TOTAL Ca= Fa= Pr= Cals=	Breakfast	
	Lunch	
	Dinner	

THURSDAY		Carbs | Fats | Proteins | Calories
TOTAL Ca= Fa= Pr= Cals=	Breakfast	
	Lunch	

	Dinner	

FRIDAY		*Carbs | Fats | Proteins | Calories*
TOTAL Ca= Fa= Pr= Cals=	Breakfast	
	Lunch	
	Dinner	

SATURDAY		*Carbs | Fats | Proteins | Calories*
TOTAL Ca= Fa= Pr= Cals=	Breakfast	
	Lunch	
	Dinner	

SUNDAY		*Carbs | Fats | Proteins | Calories*
TOTAL Ca= Fa= Pr= Cals=	Breakfast	
	Lunch	
	Dinner	

MONDAY		Carbs | Fats | Proteins | Calories
TOTAL Ca= Fa= Pr= Cals=	Breakfast	
	Lunch	
	Dinner	

TUESDAY		Carbs | Fats | Proteins | Calories
TOTAL Ca= Fa= Pr= Cals=	Breakfast	
	Lunch	
	Dinner	

WEDS		Carbs | Fats | Proteins | Calories
TOTAL Ca= Fa= Pr= Cals=	Breakfast	
	Lunch	
	Dinner	

THURSDAY		Carbs | Fats | Proteins | Calories
TOTAL Ca= Fa= Pr= Cals=	Breakfast	
	Lunch	

	Dinner	

FRIDAY		*Carbs	Fats	Proteins	Calories*
TOTAL Ca= Fa= Pr= Cals=	Breakfast	
	Lunch	
	Dinner	

SATURDAY		*Carbs	Fats	Proteins	Calories*
TOTAL Ca= Fa= Pr= Cals=	Breakfast	
	Lunch	
	Dinner	

SUNDAY		*Carbs	Fats	Proteins	Calories*
TOTAL Ca= Fa= Pr= Cals=	Breakfast	
	Lunch	
	Dinner	

4- Week Final Interval
12 Weeks Completed

Take time to assess your goals and progress. How is the program working for you?

Goals Set

Goals Reached

Set New Targets

Assess the last 4 week

QUICK REFERENCE OF HEALTHY KETO SNACKS

In case you get hungry between meals, here are some healthy, keto-approved snacks:

- Fatty meat or fish.
- Cheese.
- A handful of nuts or seeds.
- Cheese with olives.
- 1–2 hard-boiled eggs.
- 90% dark chocolate.
- A low-carb milk shake with almond milk, cocoa powder and nut butter.
- Full-fat yogurt mixed with nut butter and cocoa powder.
- Strawberries and cream.
- Celery with salsa and guacamole.
- Smaller portions of leftover meals.

Note: Great snacks for a keto diet include pieces of meat, cheese, olives, boiled eggs, nuts and dark chocolate.

NOTES & IDEAS

www.ingramcontent.com/pod-product-compliance
Lightning Source LLC
Chambersburg PA
CBHW071230240726

48654CB00009B/981